CW00427918

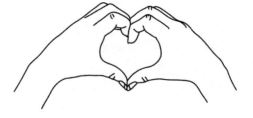

Welcome to The Little Wellness Book!

Wellness is about taking care of your body, mind and soul.

Wellness involves making small changes in your daily routine to promote well-being.

This book is a small guide that can help you on your journey towards a healthier and happier life.

On pages 35 – 42, you will find a space dedicated to journal entries. This personal section provides you with the chance to document your own reflections, dreams, and aspirations, allowing you to cultivate mindfulness, gratitude, a deeper connection with yourself, and your wellness journey.

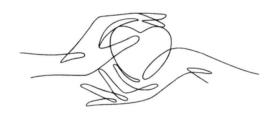

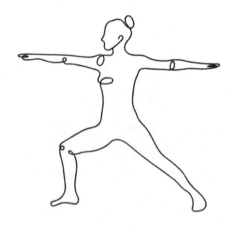

Move your body daily:

Exercise is essential for your physical and mental well-being.

Find a physical activity that you enjoy and make it a part of your daily routine.

SOME PHYSICAL EXERCISES THAT PROMOTE WELLNESS INCLUDE:

- Cardiovascular exercises, such as running, cycling, swimming, or walking, can help improve heart health, reduce the risk of chronic diseases, and promote weight loss.

- Strength training exercises, such as weightlifting or bodyweight exercises, can help improve muscle strength and tone, increase bone density, and boost metabolism.

- HIIT (High-Intensity Interval Training) workouts involve short bursts of intense exercise followed by periods of rest or low-intensity exercise. They can help improve cardiovascular fitness, increase metabolism, and promote weight loss.

- Yoga is a gentle form of exercise that can help improve flexibility, balance, and strength. It can also help reduce stress, improve sleep, and promote relaxation.

- Pilates is a low-impact exercise that can help improve core strength, flexibility, and posture. It can also help reduce stress and improve mental well-being.

- Dancing is a fun way to get moving and can help improve cardiovascular fitness, coordination, and balance. It can also help boost mood and reduce stress.

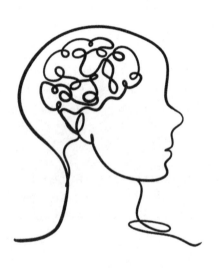

Nurture your mind:

Our mental health is just as important as our physical health.

Practice mindfulness, surround yourself with positive people and nurture your mind with positive thoughts and habits.

Incorporating mindfulness into your daily routine can help you cultivate a more positive and peaceful mindset.

Mindfulness can help reduce stress, improve focus, and promote a sense of calm and well-being.

Nourish your

Body:

Eating a balanced diet filled with fruits, vegetables, protein, and whole grains can help you maintain a healthy weight and reduce the risk of chronic diseases.

Eating well can improve your overall mental and physical well-being.

Eat well, live well.

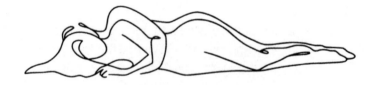

Prioritise sleep:

Sleep is essential for your overall well-being.

Aim for around 7-9 hours of sleep each night and establish a consistent sleep routine.

Sleep can improve your mood, boost your immune system, and help your body recover from the day's activities.

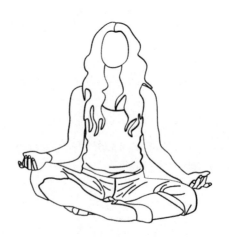

PRACTICE

STRESS-FREE

TECHNIQUES:

Stress can have a negative impact on your mental and physical health.

Regularly practicing stress-management techniques such as meditation, deep breathing, or yoga can help you manage stress levels and improve your overall well-being.

Some stress-management techniques that promote wellness include:

- Meditation: an effective technique to reduce stress.

- Deep breathing: a few deep breaths can help calm the mind and reduce stress. Take slow, deep breaths, inhaling for a count of four, holding your breath for a count of four, and exhaling for a count of four.

- Yoga: can help you manage stress levels and improve your overall well-being.

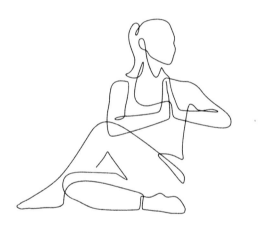

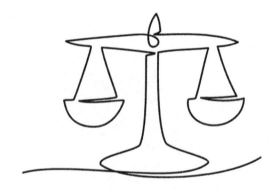

Find balance:

Finding balance is key to living a well-rounded life.

It's important to balance work and play, rest and activity, and socialising and alone time.

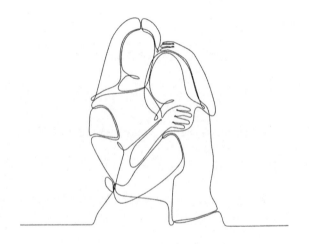

BUILD POSITIVE

RELATIONSHIPS:

Building positive relationships with family, friends, and the community can help you feel connected, supported and happy.

Social support and connection have been linked to improved physical and mental health .

SOME TECHNIQUES TO HELP BUILD POSITIVE RELATIONSHIPS FOR WELLNESS:

- Practice active listening: when socially interacting with others, try to actively listen to what they are saying. Show that you have an interest in what they have to say and respond thoughtfully.

- Practice open communication: be open and honest with the people in your life. Communicate your thoughts and feelings clearly and respectfully, and encourage them to do the same.

- Show appreciation: try to show gratitude and appreciation for the people in your life. This can be as simple as saying thank you, giving a compliment, or doing something kind for them.

- Prioritise quality time: Spend quality time with the people in your life. This can involve doing activities together, having meaningful conversations, or simply enjoying each other's company.

- Be reliable: show that you are a dependable and trustworthy person, by following through on your commitments and being there for the people in your life when they need you.

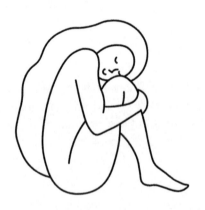

PRACTICE SELF-CARE:

Self-care is an essential component of wellness. It involves taking care of your physical, mental, and emotional health to help you feel your best.

Taking time for self-care activities such as reading, taking a peaceful bath, or spending time outdoors in nature can help you relax and recharge.

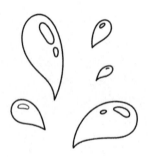

Stay hydrated:

Drinking enough water is essential for your physical and mental well-being.

Aim to drink at least 2 litres of water each day.

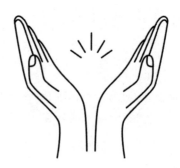

Practice

Gratitude:

Gratitude is a powerful tool for improving our overall well-being.

Cultivating a grateful mindset can improve your overall happiness.

Take time each day to reflect on the things you are grateful for.

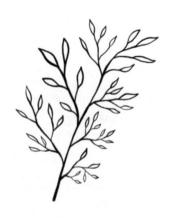

Practice

Environmental

Wellness:

Environmental wellness involves taking care of your physical environment and living in harmony with nature.

Be aware of your impact on the environment and take steps to reduce your carbon footprint; reduce waste by recycling and composting and use sustainable products and materials where possible.

Spend time in nature and appreciate the natural beauty around you.

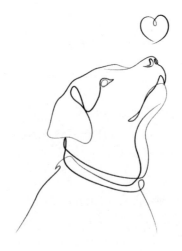

SPEND TIME WITH ANIMALS:

Spending time with animals can be incredibly beneficial for wellness.

Interacting with animals can help reduce stress, lower blood pressure, promote feelings of calm and happiness and improve overall mood.

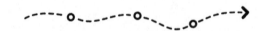

Embrace your

Journey:

Wellness is a journey that requires ongoing effort and commitment.

It is important to remember that each person's journey is unique.

Embrace your journey and enjoy the process of discovering what works best for you.

Remember that small daily changes can make a big impact on your overall happiness and well-being.

Take notes throughout your wellness journey:

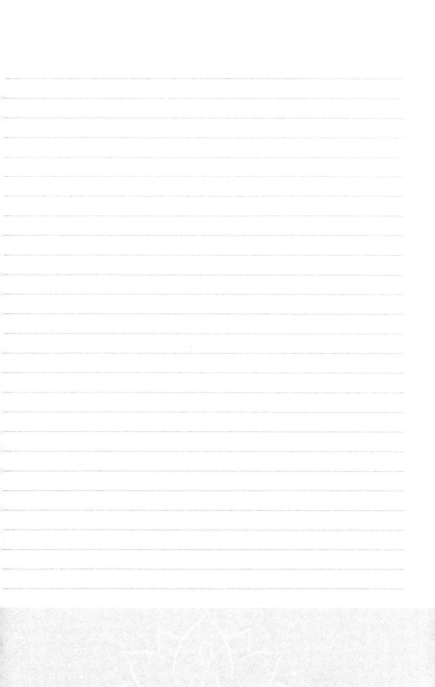

GRATITUDE LOG:

Start each day by writing down a few things you are grateful for. This can help you cultivate a positive mindset and focus on the good in your life.

MOOD LOG:

Regularly keep track of your mood. This can help you identify patterns and triggers that can affect your mood and allow you to take steps to improve your emotional well-being.

Food log:

Tracking what you eat can help you make healthier choices and identify any patterns or habits that may be affecting your nutrition.

EXERCISE LOG:

Keep track of your physical activity, logging the type of exercise,
duration, and intensity. This can help you stay motivated and track your
progress towards your fitness goals.

SLEEP LOG:

Track your sleep patterns, including the time you go to bed, the time you wake up, and the quality of your sleep. This can help you identify any factors that may be affecting your sleep and take steps to improve your sleep habits.

PRODUCTIVITY LOG:

Keep track of your daily tasks and accomplishments. This can help you stay focused and motivated, and provide a sense of satisfaction as you complete tasks and move towards your goals.

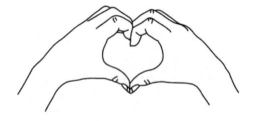

Printed in Great Britain
by Amazon